Anti Inflammatory Diet Recipes

85 Inflammation Diet Recipes

Great For Gout Relief!

Cindy Myers

I0411183

These recipes are not intended to be any type of Medical advice. ALL individuals must consult their Doctors first and should always receive their meal plans from a qualified practitioner. These recipes are not intended to heal, or cure anyone from any kind of illness, or disease.

Cream Cheese Chicken

Ratatouille with Chickpeas

Slow Cooked Chicken Fajitas

Wild Duck Breast L'Orange

Slow Roasted Herb Potatoes

Summer Squash Casserole

Caribbean Sweet Potato Stew

Slow Cooked Scalloped Potatoes

Black Bean Soup

Honey Sriracha Chicken Wings

Corn and Potato Chowder

Slow Cooked French Onion Soup

Slow Cooker Roasted Vegetables

Mix Vegetable Soup

Vermicelli with Rice

Healthy Baked Chicken

Delicious Cheese Noodles

Quick Yogurt Drink

Corn and Avocado Pasta

Sweet Potato Patties

Healthy Tofu Scrambled

Baked Zucchini with Cheese

Healthy Banana Whole Wheat Pancakes

Stuffed Banana Sandwich

Crispy Baked Zucchini

Tropical Pineapple Quinoa

Healthy Avocado Salad

Kiwi, Orange and Apple Salad

Delicious Roasted Carrots

Tropical Mango and Avocado Smoothie

Banana and Chocolate Shake

Lime and Avocado Rice

Quick and Simple Kale Salad

Stuffed Quinoa Bell Peppers

Healthy turkey Sandwich

Tasty Carrot and Sweet Potato Soup

Quick Black bean Salad

Creamy Cucumber Salad

Israeli Salad

Southwestern Egg Salad

Basil and Balsamic Mozzarella Salad

Pecan Apple Salad

Curry Chicken Salad

Chicken Basil Salad

Tuna Salad – Mediterranean

Cumin and Lime Bean Salad

Egg Salad

Barbeque Chicken Salad

Potato Summer Salad

Greek Salad

Walnut Mango Chicken Salad

Chickpea and Eggplant Salad

Tomato, Corn, and Pepper Salsa Salad

Tomato Lime Salad

Chicken Raspberry Salad

Chicken Chinese Salad

Rosemary Steak Salad

Garbanzo Bean and Salmon Salad

Grapefruit and Avocado Salad

White Bean Dip with Garlic

Vegetable Stuffed Bell Peppers

Lemon White Bean Sauce

Healthy Avocado Hummus

Easy Vegan Chili

Spicy Bean and Tofu Burger

Vanilla Mix Fruit Salad

Tangy Garlic Honey Chicken

Gluten Free Healthy Pumpkin Pancakes

Delicious Raspberry Tart

Coconut Chickpea Soup

Rosemary Lemon Chicken

Roasted Potatoes with Garlic

Mix Berries Muffins

Quick Peanut Butter Dip

Crust less Pumpkin Pie

Healthy Banana Cookies

Simple Baked Pears with Walnut

Egg less Mango Pudding

Protein Chocolate Mousse

Cucumber Salad

Avocado, Walnut and Kale Pasta

Roasted Veggies with Honey

Baked Eggplant and Zucchini with Cheese

Healthy Zucchini Hummus

Mix Berry Quinoa Breakfast

Cream Cheese Chicken

Ingredients:

3 lbs of Chicken Breast – Boneless, Skinless

1 Package of Italian Salad Dressing Mix

4 Tablespoons of Melted Butter

1 Small Onion - Chopped

1 Clove of Garlic- Chopped

1 Can of Cream of Chicken Soup

8 Ounces of Low Fat Cream Cheese

½ Cup of Chicken Broth

Instructions:

Place your chicken in your crock-pot, and then sprinkle the Italian seasoning on the chicken. Sprinkle it with 2 tablespoons of melted butter.

Cook it on the low setting for 4-6 hours.

Melt 2 tablespoons of butter in a pan, and then sauté the onions and the garlic. Add the Cream of Chicken Soup, the low fat cream cheese, as well as the chicken broth. Stir it until it is smooth.

Add the mix to your crock-pot. Cook on the low setting for an added hour.

Nutritional Information:

Calories: 547

Total Fat: 44g

Saturated Fat: 19g

Carbohydrates: 6g

Protein: 29g

Ratatouille with Chickpeas

Ingredients:

1 Tablespoon of Vegetable Oil

1 Onion - Chopped

4 Garlic Cloves - Minced

6 Cup of Eggplants - Cubed

2 Teaspoons of Basil

1 Teaspoon of Oregano

1/2 Teaspoons of Salt

1/2 Teaspoons of pepper

1 Red Bell Pepper

1 Yellow Bell Pepper

2 Zucchinis

1/3 Cups of Tomato Paste

1 Can of Chickpeas- Drained, Rinsed

1 Can of Tomatoes

1/4 Cup of Fresh Basil Chopped

Instructions:

In a large pan, heat the oil on medium, cook your onions, the garlic, the eggplant, the basil, oregano, and the salt and pepper, stirring sporadically until the onion is softened, approximately 10 minutes. Put it into the crockpot.

Halve, core, and then seed the peppers; cut them into 1-inch pieces. Cut the zucchini into halves lengthwise, and then cut them crosswise into 1 1/2-inch pieces. Add it to the crockpot.

Add tomato paste, chickpeas, and tomatoes, breaking up tomatoes with a spoon. Cover and cook on low for 4 hours, or until vegetables are tender. Stir in basil.

Nutritional Information:

Calories: 219

Total Fat: 37g

Saturated Fat: 1g

Carbohydrates: 40g

Protein: 9g

Slow Cooked Chicken Fajitas

Ingredients:

1 Red Bell Pepper

1 Yellow Bell Pepper

1 Green Bell Pepper

1 Onion

1 Packet Taco or Fajita Seasoning

1 Pound of Chicken Breasts – Boneless, Skinless

½ Cup of Chicken Broth

Toppings (Low Fat Cheese, Low Fat Sour Cream, or Salsa)

Tortillas

Instructions:

Slice the bell peppers and the onions in ¼ inch pieces. Add them to the bottom of your Crockpot.

Sprinkle the taco or fajita seasoning on the bell peppers and the onions in your Crockpot. Add in the chicken breasts and the chicken broth.

Cook it on the low setting for 6-8 hours.

Remove the chicken from the Crockpot and let cool slightly. Use two forks to shred the chicken. Add shredded chicken back to Crockpot and mix with peppers and onions.

Serve over tortillas or alone with your choice of toppings (like cheese, salsa, guacamole, sour cream, fresh cilantro).

Nutritional Information:

Calories: 235

Total Fat: 12g Saturated Fat: 7g Carbohydrates: 41g

Protein: 19g

Wild Duck Breast L'Orange

Ingredients:

2 Whole Wild Duck Breasts – Halved, Skin Removed

1/2 Teaspoons of Salt

1/4 Teaspoon of Black Pepper

2 Small Oranges – Peeled, Cut into 1/2-inch Pieces

1 Medium Apple - Cut into 1/2-inch pieces

1 Medium Onion - Cut into Eighths

1 Can (6 Ounces) Frozen Orange Juice Concentrate - Thawed

Instructions:

Sprinkle the duck with salt and pepper. Layer the duck, the oranges, the apples and the onions in a 3 1/2 - 6 quart slow cooker. Pour the orange juice concentrate on the top. Cover it and cook it on the low setting for 8-10 hours.

Remove the duck from cooker and discard the fruit and the onion mixture.

Nutritional Information:

Calories: 206

Total Fat: 4g

Saturated Fat: 1g

Carbohydrates: 32g

Protein: 13g

Slow Roasted Herb Potatoes

Ingredients:

6 Medium potatoes

1/4 Cups of Water

1 Teaspoon of Salt

1 Teaspoon of Pepper

1 Teaspoon of Garlic Powder

1 Teaspoon of Minced Onion

1/2 Teaspoons of Dried Dill

1 Teaspoon of Italian Seasoning

1 Teaspoon of Parsley

4 Tablespoon of Butter

Instructions:

Chop your potatoes into half-moons (slice the potatos in half the long-ways, then to pieces). Place them into the crock-pot.

Add the water and then sprinkle it with all the herbs and the seasoning. Stir it to distribute the herbs evenly.

Add the butter into separate pieces on the top of your potatoes.

Cover it and cook it on the low setting for 5 hours.

Nutritional Information:

Calories: 353

Total Fat: 11g

Saturated Fat: 7g

Carbohydrates: 57g

Protein: 7g

Summer Squash Casserole

Ingredients:

9 Cup of Sliced Yellow Summer Squash (5 Medium Squashes)

1 Medium Onion - Chopped

1 Tablespoon of Butter

2 Cups of French Bread Crumbs

8 Ounces of Shredded Sharp Cheddar Cheese

2/3 Cups of Low Fat Sour Cream

½ Teaspoon of Garlic Salt

¼ Teaspoon of Pepper

1 Can (10 3/4 oz) Condensed Cream of Chicken Soup

1 Tablespoon of Butter - Melted

Chopped Fresh Parsley

Instructions:

Spray a 5- to 6-quart slow cooker. In a large microwavable bowl, microwave the squash, the onion, and 1 tablespoon of butter (uncovered) on the High setting for 10 minutes. Drain it.

In your slow cooker, mix in the squash mixture, 8 ounces of the breadcrumbs, and 1/2 cup of the cheese, the low fat sour cream, the garlic salt, the pepper and the soup. In small bowl, mix remaining 8 ounces of breadcrumbs, remaining 1/2 cup of cheese and the melted butter. Sprinkle the crumb mixture over squash.

Cover it and then cook it on the low setting for 2 hours. Uncover it and remove the insert from your slow cooker. Let it stand for 30 minutes before serving. Sprinkle with parsley, if desired.

Nutritional Information:

Calories: 180

Total Fat: 12g

Saturated Fat: 6g

Carbohydrates: 12g

Protein: 5g

Caribbean Sweet Potato Stew

Ingredients:

2 Medium Sweet Potatoes

2 Chicken Breast Halves - Boneless

1 Pound of Chorizo Sausage

1 Large Onion - Chopped

2 Cloves of Garlic - Finely Minced

1 Can of Whole Tomatoes with Juice

1 Can of Garbanzo Beans - Drained

1 Teaspoon of Paprika

1 Teaspoon of Salt

1 Teaspoon of Thyme

1 Teaspoon of Ground Black Pepper

1/2 Teaspoons of Allspice

1/2 Teaspoons of Cumin

2 Tablespoons of Tomato Paste

Chopped Parsley

Instructions:

Peel and then dice the sweet potatoes into 1-inch cubes. Cut the chicken and the sausage into 1-inch pieces.

In your crock-pot, combine the sweet potatoes, your chicken, onion, sausage, garlic, tomatoes, paprika, beans, pepper, thyme, salt, allspice, the cumin, and the tomato paste. Cover it and allow it to simmer on the low setting until the sweet potatoes are tender, approximately 4 hours.

To serve it ladle it into bowls and garnish it with parsley.

Nutritional Information:

Calories: 396

Total Fat: 40g

Saturated Fat: 3g

Carbohydrates: 30g

Protein: 30g

Slow Cooked Scalloped Potatoes

Ingredients:

3 Pounds of Yukon Gold Potatoes – Unpeeled, Thinly Sliced

1 Large Onion - Thinly Sliced

1 Can of Campbell Condensed Cheddar Cheese Soup

1/2 Cups of Milk

1/2 Cups of Parmesan Cheese

1/2 Teaspoons of Salt

1/4 Teaspoon of Black Pepper

8 Ounces of Shredded Cheddar Cheese

Directions:

Spray your 6-quart slow cooker with cooking spray. Layer 1/3 of your potatoes and ½ of the onions in your cooker. Repeat layers. Top it with the rest of the potatoes.

Stir in the soup, milk, Parmesan, salt, and the black pepper in a bowl. Pour the soup mix on the potatoes. Cover it and cook it on the high setting for 4-5 hours.

Sprinkle it with Cheddar cheese. Cover it and allow it to stand for 5 minutes.

Nutritional Information:

Calories: 330

Total Fat: 11g

Saturated Fat: 6g

Carbohydrates: 46g

Protein: 12g

Black Bean Soup

Ingredients:

2 Cloves of Garlic

1 Medium Onion

2 Stalks of Celery

2 Medium Carrots

1 lb. of Black Beans - Uncooked

8 Ounces of Salsa

1 Tablespoon of Chili Powder

½ Tablespoon of Cumin

1 Tablespoon of Oregano

4 Cups of Vegetable Broth

2 Cups of Water

Instructions:

Mince the garlic, dice the onions, as well as the celery. Grate your carrots on a large cheese grater. Rinse the black beans using a colander under cold water and pick out any debris.

Combine the garlic, your onion, the celery, black beans, carrots, salsa, chili powder, oregano, cumin, the vegetable broth, and the water in your 5-7 quart cooker. Stir it well.

Place the lid on your slow cooker and then cook it on the high setting for 6-8 hours. Once the beans are soft, blend in the soup until it's thick.

Nutritional Information:

Calories: 114

Total Fat: 1g Saturated Fat: 1g

Carbohydrates: 19g

Protein: 6g

Honey Sriracha Chicken Wings

Ingredients:

4 Pounds of Chicken Wings - Frozen

3/4 Cups of Sriracha Sauce

3/4 Cups of Honey

2 Tablespoons of Unsalted Butter

Juice of One Lime

Instructions:

Add the sriracha, honey, butter, and lime juice. Stir in to combine. Add in the chicken wings. Stir it until the wings are well coated. Cook them on the low setting for 6-8 hours or on the high setting for 3-4 hours.

Remove the wings from your slow cooker and then place them on a baking sheet that is lined with foil. Drizzle on the sauce from the cooker on the wings.

Set your oven to broil. Place the baking sheet inside the oven and bake them for 2-3 minutes. Remove them from the oven.

Nutritional Information:

Calories: 321

Total Fat: 10g

Saturated Fat: 2g

Carbohydrates: 19g

Protein: 35g

Corn and Potato Chowder

Ingredients:

24 Ounces of Red Potatoes - Diced

1 (16-ounce) Package of Frozen Corn

3 Tablespoon of Flour

6 Cups of Chicken Stock

1 Teaspoon of Dried Thyme

1 Teaspoon of Dried Oregano

1/2 Teaspoons of Garlic Powder

1/2 Teaspoons of Onion Powder

Salt and Black Pepper

2 Tablespoons of Unsalted Butter

1/4 Cups of Heavy Cream

Instructions:

Place the potatoes and the corn into your slow cooker. Stir in the flour and toss it to combine it. Stir in the chicken stock, the thyme, garlic powder, oregano, onion powder, salt and pepper.

Cover it and cook it on the low setting for 7-8 hours or high heat for 3-4 hours. Stir in the butter and the heavy cream.

Serve it immediately.

Nutritional Information:

Calories: 384

Total Fat: 144g

Saturated Fat: 5g

Carbohydrates: 54g

Protein: 9g

Slow Cooked French Onion Soup

Ingredients:

1/4 Cups of Butter

6 Thyme Sprigs

1 Bay Leaf

5 Pounds of Sweet Onions - Vertically Sliced

1 Tablespoon of Sugar

6 Cups of Beef Stock

2 Tablespoons of Red Wine Vinegar

1 1/2 Teaspoons of Salt

1 Teaspoon of Black Pepper

24 Slices Whole-Grain French Bread

5 Ounces of Gruyère Cheese - Shredded

Instructions:

1. Place the butter, thyme, and the bay leaf in the bottom of your 6-quart slow cooker. Add in the onions, and then sprinkle it with sugar. Cover it and cook then cook it on the high setting for 8 hours.

2. Remove the thyme and the bay leaf; discard it. Add in the stock, vinegar, the salt, and some pepper; cook it covered on the high setting for 30 minutes.

3. Preheat your broiler to high.

4. Arrange the bread in a single layer; broil it for 30 seconds on each side. Place 8 ounces of soup on each of the12 ramekins or ovenproof bowls. Top each serving with 2 slices and 2 tablespoons of cheese. Place the 6 ramekins on a jelly-roll pan; broil it for 2 minutes or until cheese melts. Repeat the procedure with the remaining 6 ramekins, slices, and the cheese.

Nutritional Information:

Calories: 240

Total Fat: 8g

Saturated Fat: 3g

Carbohydrates: 33g

Protein: 9g

Slow Cooker Roasted Vegetables

Ingredients:

4 Potatoes – Chopped, Large Pieces

2 Carrots

1/2 Onion - Sliced

2 Zucchinis - Thickly Sliced

Olive Oil

1 Packet of Dry Italian Dressing Mix

Instructions:

Place the chopped vegetables in a bowl

Drizzle the vegetables with the olive oil.

Sprinkle the packet of Italian seasoning on the vegetables.

Lightly toss it so all of the vegetables are covered in oil and the seasoning.

Spray the slow cooker with non-stick spray and dump the seasoned vegetables in.

Cook it on the low setting for 5-7 hours or on the high setting for 3-4 hours.

Nutritional Information:

Calories: 93

Total Fat: 5g

Saturated Fat: 1g

Carbohydrates: 12g

Protein: 3g

Mix Vegetable Soup

Serves: 8

Preparation Time: 1 hour 20 minutes

Ingredients:

- 1 medium carrot, peeled and cut into small pieces
- 2 medium potato, peeled and diced into cubes
- 1 large onion, chopped
- 2 large tomatoes, chopped
- 1 cup coriander leaves, chopped
- 2 garlic clove, minced
- 1 tablespoon grated ginger
- 4 tablespoons olive oil
- 1 teaspoon pepper
- 1 teaspoon cumin
- 5 cups water
- 2 teaspoons salt

Directions:

1. Take a saucepan and heat olive oil in pan.

2. Add onion, ginger, garlic and carrots in pan and stir-fry for 5 minutes over medium heat.

3. Add tomatoes, potatoes and chopped coriander then stir-fry for further 5 minutes.

4. Add remaining ingredients and bring to boil.

5. Cover pan with lid and simmer over medium-low heat for 60 minutes. Add more water if necessary.

6. Puree soup with blender until completely smooth.

7.   Serve hot and enjoy.

Nutritional Value (Amount per Serving):

*   Calories 125

*   Fat 7.3 g

*   Saturated Fat 1 g

*   Carbohydrates 14.7 g

*   Sugar 2.9 g

*   Protein 2 g

*   Cholesterol 0 mg

Vermicelli with Rice

Serves: 4

Preparation Time: 45 minutes

Ingredients:

- 1 cup rice, rinsed
- 1/2 cup thin vermicelli, cut into small pieces
- 2 cups boiling water
- 4 tablespoons butter
- 1/4 teaspoon cinnamon
- 1/4 teaspoon pepper
- 3/4 teaspoon salt

Directions:

1. In a pan, add butter when butter melted adds vermicelli and sauté until the vermicelli pieces begin to turn golden brown.

2. Add rice in pan and stir-fry for 2 minutes.

3. Add remaining ingredients in pan except cinnamon, and then bring to boil.

4. Cover pan with lid and cook over low heat for 10 minutes.

5. Turn off heat and stir. Recover with lid and allow to cook in own steam for 25 minutes.

6. Place in serving bowl and sprinkle with cinnamon and serve with vegetable stew.

Nutritional Value (Amount per Serving):

- Calories 271
- Fat 11.8 g Saturated Fat 7.4 g
- Carbohydrates 37.2 g
- Protein 3.4 g

Healthy Baked Chicken

Serves: 2

Preparation Time: 30 minutes

Ingredients:

- 2 chicken breasts, skinless and boneless
- 1/4 cup chicken broth
- 1 1/2 tablespoons butter
- 1/2 tablespoon honey
- 2 tablespoons lemon juice
- 1/2 teaspoon Italian seasoning
- 1 teaspoon garlic, minced
- 1/4 teaspoon pepper
- 1/2 teaspoon salt

Directions:

1. Preheat your oven at 400 F and spray the baking dish with non-stick cooking spray.

2. Melt the butter in a large pan over medium high heat and add chicken breasts in pan cook chicken for 3 minutes on each side.

3. Transfer chicken in baking dish.

4. In a small bowl add lemon juice, honey, Italian seasoning, chicken broth, garlic, pepper and salt whisk together until combined.

5. Pour sauce over chicken breasts and bake for 30 minutes or until chicken cooked.

6. Garnish with lemon slices and serve.

Nutritional Value (Amount per Serving):

- Calories 376
- Fat 19.8 g
- Saturated Fat 8.6 g
- Carbohydrates 5.5 g
- Sugar 4.8 g
- Protein 42 g
- Cholesterol 150 mg

Delicious Cheese Noodles

Serves: 4

Preparation Time: 25 minutes

Ingredients:

- 1 cup parmesan cheese, grated
- 1 pound noodles
- 2 garlic cloves, minced
- 6 tablespoons canola oil
- 4 tablespoons coriander, chopped
- 1/2 teaspoon pepper
- 3/4 teaspoon salt

Directions:

1. Cook the noodles according to the directions of package.
2. Drain and place in serving bowl.
3. Add grated cheese, garlic, oil, coriander, pepper and salt in bowl and toss well until combined.
4. Serve warm and enjoy.

Nutritional Value (Amount per Serving):

- Calories 345
- Fat 23.4 g
- Saturated Fat 2 g
- Carbohydrates 29.2 g
- Protein 5.3 g
- Cholesterol 33 mg

Quick Yogurt Drink

Serves: 6

Preparation Time: 10 minutes

Ingredients:

- 4 cups low-fat yogurt
- 2 cups water
- 6 mint leaves, chopped
- Crushed ice
- 1 teaspoon salt

Directions:

1. Add yogurt, water and salt in a blender and blend for 2 minute.

2. Pour drink in serving glass and add crushed ice.

3. Garnish with chopped mint leaves. Serve immediately and enjoy.

Nutritional Value (Amount per Serving):

- Calories 116
- Fat 2 g
- Saturated Fat 1.6 g
- Carbohydrates 11.5 g
- Sugar 11.5 g
- Protein 9.3 g
- Cholesterol 10 mg

Corn and Avocado Pasta

Serves: 4

Preparation Time: 20 minutes

Ingredients:

- 1/2 cup canned corn, drained and rinsed
- 2 avocados, halved and peeled
- 12 ounces spaghetti
- 1 cup cherry tomatoes, halved
- 1/2 cup basil leaves
- 2 garlic cloves
- 2 tablespoons lemon juice
- 1/4 cup olive oil
- Pepper
- Salt

Directions:

1. Cook pasta according to the directions of package and drain well.

2. Add avocados, garlic, lemon juice, basil and olive oil in blender and blend until get smooth paste.

3. In a large bowl, add pasta, avocado paste, corn and cherry tomatoes combined well.

4. Season with pepper and salt.

5. Serve immediately and enjoy.

Nutritional Value (Amount per Serving):

- Calories 586
- Fat 34 g Saturated Fat 5.2 g Carbohydrates 60.4 g
- Protein 10.7

Sweet Potato Patties

Serves: 8

Preparation Time: 20 minutes

Ingredients:

- 2 eggs
- 2 large sweet potatoes, grated and dried
- 1/2 cup breadcrumbs
- 2 tablespoon olive oil
- 1/2 cup flour
- 1/2 teaspoon ground cinnamon
- 1/2 teaspoon salt

Directions:

1. In a bowl, add sweet potato, flour, eggs, breadcrumbs, cinnamon and salt mix well until combined.

2. Let the mixture rest for 10 minutes.

3. Heat the oil in large pan over medium heat.

4. Form the mixture into small round patties and cook patties in pan for 2 minutes on one side.

5. Turn and cook for 2 minutes until both sides are golden brown.

6. Let cool for 5 min and serve with sauce.

Nutritional Value (Amount per Serving):

- Calories 71
- Fat 1.5 g
- Carbohydrates 11
- Protein 3.1 g

Healthy Tofu Scrambled

Serves: 2

Preparation Time: 15 minutes

Ingredients:

- 14 oz tofu
- 1/2 cup onion, chopped
- 1 garlic clove, minced
- 1/4 red bell pepper, chopped
- 2 teaspoon olive oil
- 2 tablespoon chicken style seasoning
- 1/8 teaspoon turmeric powder
- Salt

Directions:

1. In a pan, add 1 teaspoon olive oil over medium heat and add chopped onion, garlic and bell pepper sauté for 3 minutes or until onion color change.

2. Set pan mixture aside.

3. In a bowl, crumbled tofu and mix chicken seasoning.

4. In another pan add remaining olive oil when oil heated, add turmeric powder.

5. Now add crumbled tofu in pan and stir continue for 3 minutes over medium heat.

6. Gently fold onion and pepper mixture in tofu and serve hot.

Nutritional Value (Amount per Serving):

- Calories 198
- Fat 13 g
- Saturated Fat 2.4 g
- Carbohydrates 7.5 g
- Sugar 2.8 g
- Protein 16.7 g
- Cholesterol 0 mg

Baked Zucchini with Cheese

Serves: 6

Preparation Time: 45 minutes

Ingredients:

- 2 cups low fat cheese
- 1/2 cup Parmesan cheese, grated
- 2 medium zucchini, sliced
- 2 tablespoons green onion, chopped
- 2 medium yellow squash, sliced
- 4 tablespoon basil, chopped
- 1/2 teaspoon dried thyme
- 3/4 teaspoon garlic powder
- Pepper
- Salt

Directions:

1. Preheat the oven at 350F and spray 8"*8" baking dish with non-stick cooking spray.

2. Combined all ingredients except Parmesan cheese and put mixture in baking dish.

3. Sprinkle grated Parmesan cheese over the top of mixture.

4. Bake uncover for 30 minutes or until zucchini cooked.

5. Serve hot and enjoy.

Nutritional Value (Amount per Serving):

- Calories 90
- Fat 2.9 g
- Saturated Fat 1.7 g
- Carbohydrates 5.6 g
- Sugar 2.6 g
- Protein 10.9 g
- Cholesterol 8 mg

Healthy Banana Whole Wheat Pancakes

Serves: 12

Preparation Time: 20 minutes

Ingredients:

- 1 egg
- 1 1/4 cup milk
- 2 ripe bananas, mashed
- 1 1/2 cups whole wheat flour
- 2 teaspoons baking powder
- 1 teaspoon vanilla
- 2 tablespoons brown sugar

Directions:

1. In a bowl, add flour, baking powder and brown sugar and mix well.

2. In another bowl whisk together egg, vanilla and milk.

3. Add wet mixture in dry mixture and stir well until combined. Fold mixture in mashed bananas.

4. Heat a non-stick pan over medium heat.

5. Add 2 tablespoon of batter over the pan and spread evenly.

6. Cook pancake for 3 minutes. Then turn another side and cook another 1 minute.

7. Make sure underside is golden brown. Repeat same with remaining batter.

8. Transfer pancake in serving plate and serve with honey and banana slice.

Nutritional Value (Amount per Serving):

- Calories 100
- Fat 1.1 g
- Carbohydrates 19.6 g
- Sugar 5.1 g
- Protein 3.1 g
- Cholesterol 16 mg

Stuffed Banana Sandwich

Serves: 2

Preparation Time: 25 minutes

Ingredients:

- 1 egg
- 4 slices of whole grain bread
- 1 large banana, peeled and sliced
- 1/4 cup milk
- 1/2 cup pecan nuts, chopped
- 1 cup cornflakes, crushed
- 1 tablespoon butter
- 1/4 teaspoon cinnamon
- 1/4 teaspoon vanilla extract

Directions:

1. Combine pecan nut and crushed cornflakes in plate and set aside.

2. Place banana slices among 2 bread slices of bread and then top with remaining bread slices to make 2 sandwiches.

3. In a bowl, add egg, vanilla, milk and whisk together until mix.

4. Dip sandwiches one by one in egg mixture and then roll in cornflakes mixture until completely coated.

5. Melt butter in pan over medium-high heat. Place sandwiches to the pan and cook each side for 2 minutes or until sandwiches are golden brown.

6. Serve immediately and enjoy.

Nutritional Value (Amount per Serving):

- Calories 340
- Fat 10.8 g
- Saturated Fat 5.3 g
- Carbohydrates 54.5 g
- Sugar 14.5 g
- Protein 11.6 g
- Cholesterol 90 mg

Crispy Baked Zucchini

Serves: 6

Preparation Time: 30 minutes

Ingredients:

- 1 cup Parmesan cheese, grated
- 6 zucchini, cut into wedges
- 4 tablespoon olive oil
- 1/2 teaspoon garlic powder
- 1 teaspoon dried thyme
- 1 teaspoon dried oregano
- 4 tablespoon chopped parsley
- Pepper
- Salt

Directions:

1. Preheat your oven at 350 F. Spray baking tray with non-stick cooking spray and set aside.

2. In a bowl, combine grated cheese, oregano, thyme, garlic powder, pepper and salt.

3. Place zucchini on baking tray and drizzle with olive oil.

4. Sprinkle cheese mixture over the zucchini and place baking tray into oven bake for 15 minutes or until crisp.

5. Garnish with chopped parsley and serve immediately.

Nutritional Value (Amount per Serving):

- Calories 114
- Fat 9.7 g
- Saturated Fat 1.4 g
- Carbohydrates 7.2 g
- Sugar 3.5 g
- Protein 2.5 g
- Cholesterol 0 mg

Tropical Pineapple Quinoa

Serves: 6

Preparation Time: 15 minutes

Ingredients:

- 2 cup fresh pineapple, diced
- 1 cup quinoa
- 1/4 cup basil leaves
- 10 ounce green giant sautés coconut packages
- 1 teaspoon red chili paste
- 2 teaspoons sugar
- 1 tablespoon oyster sauce
- 2 tablespoons soy sauce
- 2 cups water

Directions:

1. In a sauce pan, add 2 cups water and cook quinoa according to the directions of package. Set aside.

2. In small bowl, combine soy sauce, oyster sauce, sugar and red chili paste and set aside.

3. In a pan, sauté green giant coconut according to package instructions.

4. Add pineapple, cooked quinoa and basil in pan and stir constantly for 3 minutes.

5. Serve immediately and enjoy.

Nutritional Value (Amount per Serving):

- Calories 143
- Fat 1.9 g
- Saturated Fat 0 g
- Carbohydrates 27.6 g
- Sugar 7.1 g
- Protein 4.7 g
- Cholesterol 0 mg

Healthy Avocado Salad

Serves: 2

Preparation Time: 30 minutes

Ingredients:

- 1 avocado, halved, seeded and diced
- 1/4 cup basil leaves
- 1 cup cherry tomatoes, halved
- 6 cups lettuce, chopped
- 2 chicken breasts, boneless and skinless
- 6 ounces mozzarella cheese, crumbled
- 1 tablespoon olive oil
- 2 tablespoons brown sugar
- 1/2 cup balsamic vinegar
- Pepper
- Salt

Directions:

1.	In a small pan, add balsamic vinegar and brown sugar over medium heat for 6 minutes and set aside. Let it cool.

2.	Heat olive oil in pan over medium-high heat. Place chicken breast in pan and season with pepper and salt.

3.	Cook chicken for 4 minutes per side and cut into bite-size pieces.

4.	In a large bowl, place lettuce leaves and top with mozzarella cheese, chicken, avocado, basil and tomatoes.

5.	Pour balsamic vinegar and brown sugar mixture in bowl and toss well until combine.

6.   Serve immediately and enjoy.

Nutritional Value (Amount per Serving):

*   Calories 570

*   Fat 39 g

*   Saturated Fat 14 g

*   Carbohydrates 28 g

*   Sugar 12 g

*   Protein 26 g

*   Cholesterol 42 mg

Kiwi, Orange and Apple Salad

Serves: 10

Preparation Time: 15 minutes

Ingredients:

- 8 oranges, peeled and segmented
- 4 kiwis, peeled and diced
- 4 apples, diced
- 4 banana, peeled sliced
- 1 cup pomegranate
- 2 teaspoon poppy seeds
- 3 tablespoons honey
- 3 tablespoons sugar, granulated
- 1/4 cup olive oil
- 3 tablespoons lemon juice

Directions:

1.   In a small bowl, add lemon juice and sugar and whisk together until sugar dissolved.

2.   Then add olive oil, poppy seeds and honey mix well.

3.   In large bowl, add all fruits and pour lemon juice mixture over the top of fruits.

4.   Toss gently until well coated.

5.   Serve immediately and enjoy.

Nutritional Value (Amount per Serving):

- Calories 248
- Fat 6 g
- Saturated Fat 0.9 g
- Carbohydrates 51 g
- Sugar 37 g
- Protein 2.6 g
- Cholesterol 0 mg

Delicious Roasted Carrots

Serves: 4

Preparation Time: 40 minutes

Ingredients:

- 16 Ounces carrots, peeled and cut into 1 1/2 inch pieces
- 1 tablespoon thyme
- 2 tablespoons chopped parsley
- 1 tablespoon apple cider vinegar
- 3 tablespoons honey
- 3 tablespoons olive oil
- Pepper
- Salt

Directions:

1. Preheat your oven at 400 F. Spray baking tray with non-stick cooking spray.

2. Place carrots in baking tray and drizzle with olive oil.

3. Season with pepper and salt.

4. Place baking tray in oven at bake for 20 minutes.

5. In a small bowl, add vinegar and honey. Drizzle honey and vinegar mixture over the carrots and toss well.

6. Place baking tray again in oven and bake for 15 minutes.

7. Remove tray from oven and sprinkle with thyme and chopped parsley toss well and serve.

Nutritional Value (Amount per Serving):

- Calories 188
- Fat 10.6 g
- Saturated Fat 1.5 g
- Carbohydrates 24.7 g
- Sugar 18.6 g
- Protein 1.1 g
- Cholesterol 0 mg

Tropical Mango and Avocado Smoothie

Serves: 6

Preparation Time: 15 minutes

Ingredients:

- 1 ripe avocado, peeled and cored
- 2 kiwis, peeled
- 2 cups pineapple juice
- 2 cup mango chunks
- 2 cup strawberries
- 1 cup coconut milk

Directions:

1. Pour pineapple juice in blender and add mangoes, avocado and kiwis and blend until smooth.

2. Pour mixture into 6 glasses.

3. Then add coconut milk and strawberries in blender and blend until smooth.

4. Spoon coconut milk and strawberry mixture in glasses.

5. Serve immediately and enjoy.

Nutritional Value (Amount per Serving):

- Calories 235
- Fat 16.4 g
- Saturated Fat 9 g
- Carbohydrates 23 g
- Sugar 14 g
- Protein 2.5 g
- Cholesterol 0 mg

Banana and Chocolate Shake

Serves: 2

Preparation Time: 10 minutes

Ingredients:

* 2 tablespoons coco powder
* 2 ripe bananas, peeled and sliced
* 1/2 teaspoon vanilla extract
* 1/4 cup peanut butter, creamy
* 1 cup ice
* 1 cup almond milk

Directions:

1. Add all ingredients in blender and blend until get smooth mixture.

2. Pour in the glasses and serve immediately.

Nutritional Value (Amount per Serving):

* Calories 572
* Fat 42 g
* Saturated Fat 28 g
* Carbohydrates 39 g
* Sugar 19 g
* Protein 12 g
* Cholesterol 0 mg

Lime and Avocado Rice

Serves: 4

Preparation Time: 15 minutes

Ingredients:

- 2 ripe avocado, peeled and cored
- 4 cups brown rice, cooked
- 1 garlic clove, minced
- 1/4 teaspoon ground cumin
- 1/4 cup cilantro, chopped
- 2 tablespoon lime juice
- Pepper
- Salt

Directions:

1. In a large bowl, mashed avocados.
2. Add lemon juice, cumin, garlic and chopped cilantro in bowl and mix well.
3. Season with avocados mixture with pepper and salt.
4. Stir avocados mixture in warm rice and serve immediately.

Nutritional Value (Amount per Serving):

- Calories 842
- Fat 20 g
- Saturated Fat 4.3 g
- Carbohydrates 142 g
- Sugar 0.6 g
- Protein 15.9 g
- Cholesterol 0 mg

Quick and Simple Kale Salad

Serves: 6

Preparation Time: 15 minutes

Ingredients:

- 1/2 cup parmesan cheese, grated
- 2 bunch of kale, steams removed
- 1 teaspoon Dijon mustard
- 2 garlic cloves, minced
- 1/4 cup olive oil
- 2 tablespoons lemon juice
- 1/2 cup almonds
- Pepper
- Salt

Directions:

1. Cut the kale into bite size pieces.
2. In a small bowl, add mustard, garlic, olive oil, lemon juice, pepper and salt mix well.
3. In a large mixing bowl, Add kale leaves, almonds and grated cheese mix well until combined.
4. Pour dressing over the top of kale salad and toss well until evenly coated.
5. Serve immediately and enjoy.

Nutritional Value (Amount per Serving):

- Calories 121
- Fat 12.4 g Saturated Fat 1.5 g Carbohydrates 2.2 g
- Protein 1.8 g

Stuffed Quinoa Bell Peppers

Serves: 2

Preparation Time: 40 minutes

Ingredients:

- 2 red bell peppers, cut into half
- 1/2 cup quinoa, cooked
- 1/4 teaspoon olive oil
- 1 tablespoon lemon juice
- 1 garlic clove, minced
- 1/2 cup goat cheese, crumbled
- 1 cup cherry tomatoes, quartered
- 8 ounce asparagus, trimmed and cut into 1/4" pieces
- Pepper
- Salt

Directions:

1. Preheat your oven at 400 F.

2. Spray baking tray with non-stick cooking spray.

3. Place bell peppers on baking tray. Drizzle with olive oil and season with pepper and salt.

4. Place baking tray in oven and bake for 15 minutes. Remove tray from oven and set aside.

5. In a bowl, add cooked quinoa, lemon juice, garlic, olive oil and pepper mix well until combined.

6. Add cherry tomatoes and asparagus in quinoa bowl. Mix well.

7. Stuffed quinoa in bell peppers halves and place crumbled cheese over the top of each pepper.

8. Place stuffed peppers in oven and bake for 5 minutes until cheese is softened.

9. Serve immediately and enjoy.

Nutritional Value (Amount per Serving):

- Calories 242
- Fat 3.9 g
- Saturated Fat 0.6 g
- Carbohydrates 42 g
- Sugar 9.7 g
- Protein 10.6 g
- Cholesterol 0 mg

Healthy turkey Sandwich

Serves: 2

Preparation Time: 20 minutes

Ingredients:

- 16 ounce roasted turkey breast, cut into pieces
- 2 slices tomato
- 2 slices lettuce
- 1 avocado, mashed
- 4 slices whole grain bread
- 1/4 cup cilantro
- 1 teaspoon chili powder
- 1 teaspoon cumin
- 1/4 cup chopped onion
- 1 cup cottage cheese
- 1 can black beans, drained
- 1 garlic clove
- Salt

Directions:

1. Add garlic, black beans, cheese, onion, cumin, chili powder, cilantro and salt in blender and blend until get smooth paste.

2. Spread black bean paste onto two slices of bread then spread avocado mashed remaining bread slices.

3. Place turkey, tomatoes and lettuce over the top of black bean spread bread slices.

4. Cover the sandwiches with avocado spread bread slices.

5. Serve immediately and enjoy.

Nutritional Value (Amount per Serving):

- Calories 456
- Fat 24 g
- Saturated Fat 5.4 g
- Carbohydrates 41 g
- Sugar 6 g
- Protein 24 g
- Cholesterol 9 mg

Tasty Carrot and Sweet Potato Soup

Serves: 4

Preparation Time: 35 minutes

Ingredients:

- 16 ounce sweet potatoes, peeled and cut into chunks
- 10 ounce carrots, peeled and cut into chunks
- 4 cups vegetable stock
- 3/4 cup cream
- 2 garlic clove, minced
- 2 onions, chopped
- 3 tablespoon olive oil
- Pepper
- Salt

Directions:

1. Heat oven at 200 F. Place carrots and sweet potatoes onto the roasting tray and drizzle with 2 tbsp olive oil and season with pepper and salt.

2. Place tray in oven and roast for 25 minutes or until carrots and potatoes are tender.

3. In a sauce pan, add 1 tablespoon olive oil over the medium-high heat.

4. Add onion in pan sauté it for 10 minutes. Then add garlic and vegetable stock.

5. Remove roasted vegetables from oven and leave it to little cool.

6.   Now add roasted vegetables in sauce pan and blend it with hand blender until get smooth mixture.

7.   Stir cream in sauce and serve hot.

Nutritional Value (Amount per Serving):

- Calories 306
- Fat 13 g
- Saturated Fat 3.1 g
- Carbohydrates 45 g
- Sugar 7.3 g
- Protein 3.4 g
- Cholesterol 8 mg

Quick Black bean Salad

Serves: 4

Preparation Time: 15 minutes

Ingredients:

- 1 can black beans, drained and rinsed
- 2 tablespoon lemon juice
- 2 tablespoon chopped cilantro
- 1/2 bell pepper, chopped
- 8 ounce can corn, drained and rinsed
- Pepper
- Salt

Directions:

1.   In a mixing bowl, add beans, chopped pepper, cilantro and corn. Mix well until combined.

2.   Drizzle with lemon juice and season with pepper and salt.

3.   Toss salad gently to blend.

4.   Chilled salad in refrigerator for 30 minutes before serving.

5.   Serve chilled and enjoy.

Nutritional Value (Amount per Serving):

- Calories 53
- Fat 0.6 g
- Saturated Fat 0 g
- Carbohydrates 11.8 g
- Sugar 2.5 g
- Protein 1.7 g
- Cholesterol 0 mg

Creamy Cucumber Salad

Ingredients:

1 Cup of Yogurt – Low Fat

2 Tbsp. of Vinegar

2 tsp. of Sweetener

½ tsp. of Dill

1 Large Cucumber – Peeled, Sliced Thin

4 Tomatoes – Cubed

1 Green Pepper – Diced

½ Red Onion – Sliced Thin

Directions:

Stir in the yogurt, sweetener, vinegar, and the dill.

Add the pepper and the salt.

Add the tomatoes, cucumbers, peppers, and the onion. Toss it to coat.

Cover it and allow it to chill for 2-48 hours. Stir it often. Stir it before you serve it.

Nutritional Information:

Calories: 31

Total Fat: 0g

Saturated Fat: 0g

Carbohydrates: 6g

Protein: 2g

Israeli Salad

Ingredients:

2 Cucumbers

4 Tomatoes

1 Green Pepper

1 Tbsp. of Virgin Olive Oil

3 Tbsp. of Lemon Juice

Directions:

Dice all of the vegetables.

Combine all of the ingredients.

Allow it to stand for 30 minutes.

Nutritional Information:

Calories: 43

Total Fat: 2g

Saturated Fat: 0g

Carbohydrates: 7g

Protein: 1g

Southwestern Egg Salad

Ingredients:

2 Eggs – Hard Boiled

8 Egg Whites

2 Medium Scallions – Chopped Fine

1 tsp. of Green Chili Peppers – Drained, Chopped

1 Tbsp. of Cilantro – Minced

½ Small Red Pepper – Chopped Fine

¼ tsp. of Cumin

¼ tsp. of Salt

1/8 tsp. of Pepper

Directions:

Peel the eggs and mash it with a fork.

Add in the rest of the ingredients and mix it well.

Serve it in the bell pepper.

Nutritional Information:

Calories: 124

Total Fat: 7g

Saturated Fat: 1g

Carbohydrates: 6g

Protein: 10g

Basil and Balsamic Mozzarella Salad

Ingredients:

2 Medium Tomatoes – Peeled, Diced

1 Ounce of Mozzarella Cheese – Shredded

2 Green Onions – Chopped

2 Tbsp. of Red Onion – Diced

2 Tbsp. of Basil

2 Tbsp. of Balsamic Vinegar

1 tsp. Italian Seasoning

1 Clove of Garlic – Minced

Directions:

Mix all of the ingredients together.

Let it sit for at least 10 minutes.

Nutritional Information:

Calories: 86

Total Fat: 4g

Saturated Fat: 2g

Carbohydrates: 10g

Protein: 5g

Pecan Apple Salad

Ingredients:

8 Ounces of Avocado – Chopped

8 Ounces of Celery – Chopped

5 Large Apples – Fuji, Chopped

5 Scallions – Chopped

3 Ounces of Pecans – Chopped

14 Ounces of Chicken – Canned

2 Large Tomatoes – Chopped

2 Cucumbers – Chopped

20 Cups of Lettuce

1 Ounce of Lemon Juice

1 Ounce of Lime Juice

Directions:

Chop the first eight ingredients, and then mix them together in a large mixing bowl.

Add in the juices.

Place the mix on top of the greens.

Top it with your favorite salad dressing.

Nutritional Information:

Calories: 124

Total Fat: 7g

Saturated Fat: 1g

Carbohydrates: 6g

Protein: 10g

Curry Chicken Salad

Ingredients:

½ Cup of Cottage Cheese – Low Fat

1 tsp. of Curry Powder

Dash of Salt

Dash of Pepper

2 Spring Onions – Large

¼ Cup of Walnut Halves – Chopped

1 Small Apple – Peeled, Cubed

2 Cups of Chicken Breast – Chopped

Directions:

Puree the cottage cheese in a blender or a food processor.

Add in the curry powder, pepper, and the salt. Mix it very well.

Serve on a bed of lettuce or on a pita.

Nutritional Information:

Calories: 197

Total Fat: 7g

Saturated Fat: 1g

Carbohydrates: 6g

Protein: 6g

Chicken Basil Salad

Ingredients:

6 Tbsp. of Mayonnaise – Fat Free

2 Tbsp. of Lemon Juice

2 tsp. of Dijon Mustard

¼ tsp. of Hot Sauce

1/8 tsp. of White Pepper

3 Cups of Chicken Breasts – Chopped

½ Cup of Celery – Chopped

¼ Green Onions – Chopped

¼ Cup of Basil

6 Cups of Romaine – Shredded

Directions:

Combine your first five ingredients and mix it well.

Combine the chicken, green onions, celery, and the basil in a medium mixing bowl.

Add in the mayonnaise mix and toss it gently.

Place one cup of romaine on each plate.

Sprinkle it with pine nuts.

Nutritional Information:

Calories: 124

Total Fat: 7g

Saturated Fat: 1g

Carbohydrates: 6g

Protein: 10g

Tuna Salad – Mediterranean

Ingredients:

5 Ounces of Tuna – Light

3 Ounces of Tomatoes – Diced

¼ Avocado

1 tsp. of Virgin Olive Oil

1 Ounce of Feta Cheese – Reduced Fat

Directions:

Drain your tuna and put it in a medium bowl.

Add in ½ - 1 tablespoon of liquid that your tomatoes were packed in.

Add in 2-3 tablespoons of diced tomatoes.

Add in about one tsp. of olive oil and the diced avocado.

Crumble in the feta cheese.

Mix it all together well and be gentle.

Season it with salt and pepper.

You can let it sit overnight if you choose.

Nutritional Information:

Calories: 124

Total Fat: 7g

Saturated Fat: 1g

Carbohydrates: 6g

Protein: 10g

Cumin and Lime Bean Salad

Ingredients:

1 Can of Corn

1 Cup of Black Beans

1 Cup of Chickpeas

Juice from 3 Limes

2 Tbsp. of Virgin Olive Oil

4 Tbsp. of Cumin

Directions:

Strain all of the canned goods, and then rinse them.

Put it in a large serving bowl.

Add in the oil and cumin.

Mix it well.

Nutritional Information:

Calories: 178

Total Fat: 7g

Saturated Fat: 1g

Carbohydrates: 28g

Protein: 6g

Egg Salad

Ingredients:

3 Eggs – Boiled

8 Egg Whites – Boiled

1/3 Cup of Hellman's Light

1 tsp. of Mustard

1 Tbsp. of Pickle Relish

¼ Cup of Green Onion – Chopped

Directions:

Mix all of the ingredients.

Nutritional Information:

Calories: 124

Total Fat: 7g

Saturated Fat: 1g

Carbohydrates: 6g

Protein: 10g

Barbeque Chicken Salad

Ingredients:

4 Cups of Lettuce

½ Tomato – Sliced

½ Tbsp. of American Cheese – Shredded

1 Tbsp. of Corn

2 ½ Ounce of Chicken Breast – Skinless

Directions:

Chop your lettuce.

Add in the tomatoes and the cheese.

Add in the corn.

Cook the chicken and baste it with the barbeque.

Mix it all together.

Nutritional Information:

Calories: 124

Total Fat: 7g

Saturated Fat: 1g

Carbohydrates: 6g

Protein: 10g

Potato Summer Salad

Ingredients:

3 Pounds of Potatoes – Cut into Cubes

½ Red Onion – Sliced Thin

½ Cup of Cherry Tomatoes – Halved

¼ Cup of Bacon Bits

4 Tbsp. of Basil

¼ Cup of Italian Dressing

¼ Cup of Mayonnaise

2 tsp. of Dijon Mustard

Directions:

Cook your potatoes until they are tender. Drain them. Put them in a large mixing bowl.

Add in the onions, bacon, tomatoes, and basil.

Mix it thoroughly.

Mix in the rest of the ingredients.

Add the potato mix and toss it to coat it.

Refrigerate it for hours until it is chilled.

Nutritional Information:

Calories: 187

Total Fat: 5g

Saturated Fat: 1g

Carbohydrates: 30g

Protein: 5g

Greek Salad

Ingredients:

1 Cucumber – Diced

2 Large Tomatoes – Diced

½ Cup of Red Onion – Sliced Thin

½ Cup of Green Bell Pepper – Sliced Thin

1 Cup of Feta Cheese

2 Tbsp. of Oregano

2 tsp. of Lemon Juice

2 Tbsp. of Olive Oil

Directions:

In a medium-mixing bowl, layer it with cucumbers, onion, tomatoes, pepper, and the feta cheese.

Sprinkle it with oregano.

Drizzle it with lemon juice and the olive oil.

Season it with salt and pepper.

Nutritional Information:

Calories: 124

Total Fat: 7g

Saturated Fat: 1g

Carbohydrates: 6g

Protein: 10g

Walnut Mango Chicken Salad

Ingredients:

1 ½ Pounds of Chicken Breast – Cubed

½ Cup of Mayonnaise – Reduced Fat

1/3 Cup of Yogurt – Plain, Fat Free

5 tsp. of Curry Powder

1 Tbsp. of Lime Juice

1 tsp. of Honey

½ tsp. of Ginger – Ground

½ tsp. of Salt

¼ tsp. of Pepper

½ Cup of Red Onion – Chopped

1 Mango – Peeled

¾ Cup of Seedless Grapes – Halved

½ Cup of Walnuts – Chopped

Directions:

Chop your chicken into pieces.

Whisk the yogurt, mayonnaise, lime juice, ginger, honey, pepper, and salt in a large mixing bowl.

Add in the onion, chicken, mango, grapes, and the walnuts.

Stir it softly to combine it.

Nutritional Information:

Calories: 124

Total Fat: 7g

Saturated Fat: 1g

Carbohydrates: 6g

Protein: 10g

Chickpea and Eggplant Salad

Ingredients:

2 Eggplants – Cut lengthwise, 1 Inch Slices

½ tsp. of Salt – Divided

2 Tbsp. of Olive Oil

½ tsp. of Pepper

32 Ounces of Chickpeas, Drained, Rinsed

1 Cup of Cherry Tomatoes – Sliced

1 Tbsp. of Parsley – Chopped

2 Tbsp. of Red Wine Vinegar

2 Tbsp. of Lemon Juice

2 Cloves of Garlic – Minced

½ tsp. of Lemon Zest

Directions:

Layer a baking sheet with paper towels.

Place the eggplant on the top in a single layer.

Sprinkle it with the salt.

Cover it with paper towels.

Let the eggplant stand for at least 30 minutes.

Rinse each of the pieces and blot it dry.

Brush the sides with olive oil.

Season it with pepper.

Heat the grill to medium heat.

Grill the eggplant for 16-20 minutes; only turning once.

When the eggplant is cooled off, cut it into ½ inch cubes.

Toss the eggplant, the chickpeas, and the parsley in a large mixing bowl.

Whisk the oil, vinegar, lemon juice, garlic, and lemon zest together.

Pour it over the salad and gently toss it.

Allow it to stand for 20 minutes.

Nutritional Information:

Calories: 189

Total Fat: 8g

Saturated Fat: 1g

Carbohydrates: 23g

Protein: 6g

Tomato, Corn, and Pepper Salsa Salad

Ingredients:

1 Ear of Corn –Steamed, Cut from Cob

1 Large Tomato – Seeded, Chopped

1 Red Pepper – Roasted, Chopped

¼ Chili Pepper

2 Tbsp. of Olive Oil

2 Tbsp. of Lime Juice

Dash of Salt

Dash of Pepper

Directions:

Prepare all of your ingredients.

Allow it to stand for at least 10 minutes before you serve it.

Nutritional Information:

Calories: 124

Total Fat: 7g

Saturated Fat: 1g

Carbohydrates: 6g

Protein: 10g

Tomato Lime Salad

Ingredients:

1 ½ Cup of Tomatoes – Diced

1 Cup of Green Onions – Chopped

1 Cup of Cucumbers – Chopped

¼ Cup of Lime Juice

2 tsp. of Grapeseed Oil

4 Ounces of Green Leaf Lettuce

3 Ounces of Carrots

2 Tbsp. of Sweetener

Directions:

Mix all of the ingredients together.

Nutritional Information:

Calories: 115

Total Fat: 5g

Saturated Fat: 1g

Carbohydrates: 18g

Protein: 3g

Chicken Raspberry Salad

Ingredients:

7 Cups of Romaine Lettuce

2 Cups of Raspberries

¼ Cup of Red Onions – Sliced Thin

¼ Pound of Chicken – Boneless, Skinless

Directions:

Toss the romaine lettuce with the rest of the ingredients.

Drizzle it with the dressing.

Nutritional Information:

Calories: 111

Total Fat: 2g

Saturated Fat: 1g

Carbohydrates: 13g

Protein: 10g

Chicken Chinese Salad

Ingredients:

4 Ounces of Chicken – Boneless, Skinless, Cubed

2 Cups of Romaine Lettuce – Chopped

1 Tbsp. of Soy Sauce – Low Sodium

1 Tbsp. of Olive Oil

1 Tbsp. of Vinegar

1 tsp. of Dijon Mustard

1 Tbsp. of Sesame Seeds

Directions:

Combine all of the ingredients together.

Allow it to sit for 10 minutes.

Nutritional Information:

Calories: 124

Total Fat: 7g

Saturated Fat: 1g

Carbohydrates: 6g

Protein: 10g

Rosemary Steak Salad

Ingredients:

1/3 Cups of Red Wine Vinegar

¼ Cup of Water

3 Tbsp. of Olive Oil

2 Tbsp. of Lemon Juice

2 Cloves of Garlic – Minced

2 tsp. of Sweetener

3 Tbsp. of Rosemary

3 Tbsp. of Thyme

3 Tbsp. of Oregano

3 Tbsp. of Basil

½ tsp. of Salt

¼ tsp. of Pepper

1 Pounce of Sirloin Steak – Grilled, Fat Trimmed

1 Medium Onion

6 Medium Tomatoes – Wedges

2 Cups of Corn – Cooked

1 Medium Green Pepper – Sliced

Directions:

Grill the steak, and then slice it.

Add in all of the ingredients and mix it.

Nutritional Information:

Calories: 306

Total Fat: 13g Saturated Fat: 3g

Carbohydrates: 23g

Protein: 27g

Garbanzo Bean and Salmon Salad

Ingredients:

5 ½ Ounces of Salmon – Canned

3 Cups of Romaine

3 Cups of Iceberg Lettuce

4 Tbsp. of Lemon Juice

1 Tbsp. of Olive Oil

2 Green Onions – Diced

1 Cup of Garbanzo Beans

Directions:

Mix the beans, salmon, green onions, olive oil, and lemon juice together.

Add the salmon to the top of lettuce.

Nutritional Information:

Calories: 124

Total Fat: 7g

Saturated Fat: 1g

Carbohydrates: 6g

Protein: 10g

Grapefruit and Avocado Salad

Ingredients:

2 Grapefruits

1 Avocado

2 Tbsp. of Lime Juice

½ tsp. of Honey

1 ½ tsp. of Ginger – Grated

½ tsp. of Salt

¼ tsp. of Pepper

1 Tbsp. of Mint

1 Head of Iceberg Lettuce

Directions:

Segment your grapefruits and then drain over your mesh strainer.
Reserve the juice.

Add ¼ cup of water.

Puree juice, lime juice, ¼ of an avocado, ginger, pepper, and salt.

Pour it on the salad, and then toss it together.

Nutritional Information:

Calories: 60

Total Fat: 4g

Saturated Fat: 1g

Carbohydrates: 7g

Protein: 1g

White Bean Dip with Garlic

Serves: 2

Preparation Time: 15 minutes

Ingredients:

- 2 tablespoon garlic, roasted
- 14 ounce can white bean, drained and rinsed
- 2 tablespoon lemon juice
- 2 tablespoon olive oil
- Pepper
- Salt

Directions:

1. Place all ingredients in blender and blend until get smooth paste.

2. Season with extra seasoning if desired.

3. Serve with tortilla chips and enjoy.

Nutritional Value (Amount per Serving):

- Calories 136
- Fat 14.2 g
- Saturated Fat 2.1 g
- Carbohydrates 3.1 g
- Protein 0.7 g
- Cholesterol 0 mg

Vegetable Stuffed Bell Peppers

Serves: 4

Preparation Time: 50 minutes

Ingredients:

- 4 green bell peppers
- 1 cup wild rice, cooked
- 1 teaspoon mix herb
- 1 teaspoon chili flakes
- 1/2 teaspoon garlic powder
- 1 cup tomato sauce
- 1/2 cup corn
- 15 ounce kidney beans, cooked
- 1 onion, chopped
- 1/2 teaspoon cumin
- 2 tablespoon olive oil

Directions:

1. In a mixing bowl, combine all ingredients except olive oil and green bell pepper.

2. Preheat your oven at 350 F.

3. Spray baking tray with non-stick cooking spray.

4. Remove seeds from bell peppers.

5. Stuffed wild rice mixture in bell peppers and place onto baking tray.

6. Place baking tray in oven and bake for 35 minutes.

7. Remove from oven and serve hot.

Nutritional Value (Amount per Serving):

- Calories 639

- Fat 9.2 g

- Saturated Fat 1.3 g

- Carbohydrates 106 g

- Protein 32 g

- Cholesterol 0 mg

Lemon White Bean Sauce

Serves: 2

Preparation Time: 15 minutes

Ingredients:

- 3 cups white beans, cooked
- 2 tablespoon olive oil
- 1/2 cup water
- 1/2 cup lemon juice
- 2 tablespoon mint, dried
- 3 garlic clove, minced
- Salt

Directions:

1. In a pot, combined all ingredients over the medium heat.

2. Mash half beans mixture using back of ladle.

3. Drizzle extra olive oil over bean sauce and serve with flat bread.

Nutritional Value (Amount per Serving):

- Calories 950
- Fat 17.1 g
- Saturated Fat 3.1 g
- Carbohydrates 175 g
- Sugar 7.7 g
- Protein 71 g
- Cholesterol 0 mg

Healthy Avocado Hummus

Serves: 4

Preparation Time: 15 minutes

Ingredients:

- 2 ripe avocados, peeled and cored
- 1 can chickpea, drained
- 2 garlic clove
- 2 tablespoon olive oil
- 3 tablespoon lemon juice
- 4 tablespoon tahini
- Salt

Directions:

1.	Add chickpea, olive oil, garlic, lemon juice and tahini in blender and blend until smooth.

2.	Add 3 tablespoon water in blender mixture and blend again until get smooth and creamy mixture.

3.	Season with salt and add avocados and blend it again until creamy.

4.	Drizzle with olive oil and serve with flatbread.

Nutritional Value (Amount per Serving):

- Calories 360
- Fat 34.2 g
- Saturated Fat 6.3 g
- Carbohydrates 12.2 g
- Sugar 0.8 g
- Protein 4.2 g

Easy Vegan Chili

Serves: 6

Preparation Time: 50 minutes

Ingredients:

- 2 can tomatoes with juice
- 3 stalks celery, diced
- 2 cup corn
- 2 can kidney beans, drained and rinsed
- 2 tablespoon olive oil
- 2 teaspoon chili flakes
- 2 green peppers, diced
- 1 onion, diced
- 2 carrots, diced
- 4 garlic cloves, minced
- 1 teaspoon oregano
- 2 tablespoon chili powder
- 2 tablespoon cumin
- 1/2 cup sour cream
- Salt

Directions:

1. In a pot, add olive oil over medium-high heat add onion in pot and sauté for 4 minutes.

2. Add garlic in pot and sauté 2 minute more.

3. Add spices in pot and cook for 1 minute.

4. Add carrots, celery and pepper in pot and sauté for 5 minutes until soften.

5.   Now add tomatoes with juice in pot and reduce heat to medium-low.

6.   Stir continue and cook for 15 minutes then add beans and corn in pot and simmer for 5 minutes.

7.   Add salt as per your taste and stir.

8.   Stir in sour cream and serve hot.

Nutritional Value (Amount per Serving):

- Calories 167
- Fat 10 g
- Saturated Fat 3.4 g
- Carbohydrates 19.2 g
- Sugar 4.7 g
- Protein 3.5 g
- Cholesterol 8 mg

Spicy Bean and Tofu Burger

Serves: 4

Preparation Time: 20 minutes

Ingredients:

- 4 ounce goat cheese, crumbled
- 4 ounce soft tofu
- 1 small onion, chopped
- 1/2 bell pepper, chopped
- 8 ounce can black beans, drained and rinsed
- 1 cup arugula
- 8 burger buns
- 2 teaspoon olive oil
- 1 cup breadcrumbs
- 2 teaspoon garam masala
- Mayonnaise
- Salt

Directions:

1. Cook and mashed black beans in large bowl then add onion, pepper, garam masala and salt mix well until combined.

2. Combine tofu and breadcrumbs in patty mixture.

3. Make 4 round shape patty from mixture and set aside for 10 minutes.

4. In a pan, add olive oil over medium-high heat and place patty into the pan cook each side for 3 minutes or until golden brown.

5. Spread mayonnaise in burger bun place patty, arugula and cheese.

6. Assemble remaining burger same.

7. Serve hot and enjoy.

Nutritional Value (Amount per Serving):

- Calories 337
- Fat 15.2 g
- Saturated Fat 7.8 g
- Carbohydrates 32.2 g
- Sugar 4.4 g
- Protein 17.6 g
- Cholesterol 30 mg

Vanilla Mix Fruit Salad

Serves: 4

Preparation Time: 10 minutes

Ingredients:

- 1/2 teaspoon vanilla extract
- 2 tablespoon lemon juice
- 2 tablespoon vanilla pudding mix
- 1/2 cup strawberries, sliced
- 1 cup grapes
- 1/2 cup blueberries
- 1/2 cup pineapple chunks
- 1/2 cup raspberries

Directions:

1. In a bowl, mix all fruits.

2. Add vanilla pudding powder, vanilla extract over the top of fruits.

3. Drizzle with lemon juice and toss well until coated.

4. Serve immediately and enjoy.

Nutritional Value (Amount per Serving):

- Calories 60
- Fat 0.4 g
- Saturated Fat 0 g
- Carbohydrates 12.7 g
- Sugar 8.6 g
- Protein 0.8 g
- Cholesterol 0 mg

Tangy Garlic Honey Chicken

Serves: 4

Preparation Time: 25 minutes

Ingredients:

- 18 ounce chicken breast, boneless and skinless
- 3 tablespoon Dijon mustard
- 1/4 cup honey
- 3 garlic cloves, minced
- 2 tablespoon olive oil
- 1/4 cup parsley, chopped
- Pepper
- Salt

Directions:

1. In a pan, add 1 tbsp olive oil over medium-high heat and place chicken breasts in pan.

2. Season chicken with pepper and salt and cook for 4 minutes each side or until chicken cooked.

3. Remove chicken from pan and set aside.

4. In small bowl, combine 1 tbsp olive oil, garlic, mustard and honey.

5. Pour honey mixture over the chicken and place chicken again in pan. Cook for 3 minutes.

6. Garnish chicken with chopped parsley and serve hot.

Nutritional Value (Amount per Serving):

- Calories 347
- Fat 12.1 g Saturated Fat 1.0 g Carbohydrates 19.1 g
- Protein 41.8 g

Gluten Free Healthy Pumpkin Pancakes

Serves: 6

Preparation Time: 15 minutes

Ingredients:

- 3 eggs
- 1/4 cup pumpkin puree
- 3 tablespoon almond milk
- 1/4 teaspoon baking powder
- 1 teaspoon cinnamon
- 1/4 cup coconut flour
- 1 teaspoon vanilla
- 1 tablespoon olive oil
- 1 tablespoon honey
- 1 tablespoon vegetable oil
- Salt

Directions:

1. In a bowl, combine coconut flour, baking powder, salt and cinnamon.

2. Take one more bowl, add egg, pumpkin puree, almond milk, honey, oil and vanilla whisk together until mix.

3. Add dry ingredients in egg mixture and combined together.

4. Heat non-stick pan over medium heat. Coat pan with vegetable oil.

5. Pour 1/4 cup batter onto pan and cook for each side 4 minutes or until golden brown.

6. Repeat same with remaining batter.

7.   Serve pancakes with maple syrup and enjoy.

Nutritional Value (Amount per Serving):

*   Calories 106
*   Fat 8.6 g
*   Saturated Fat 3.1 g
*   Carbohydrates 4.8 g
*   Sugar 3.7 g
*   Protein 3.1 g
*   Cholesterol 82 mg

Delicious Raspberry Tart

Serves: 6

Preparation Time: 50 minutes

Ingredients:

- 1 egg yolk
- 1 cup raspberry jam
- 2 tablespoon butter
- 1/4 cup brown sugar
- 1/4 cup all purpose flour
- 1 cup fresh raspberries
- 1/2 teaspoon vanilla extract
- 1 stick butter salted, diced
- 1/2 teaspoon baking powder
- 1/2 cup sugar
- 1 cup all purpose flour

Directions:

1. Preheat your oven at 350 F.

2. In bowl mix flour, sugar and salt then add butter and mix until mixture becomes crumbled.

3. Now add egg and vanilla extract mix together until it forms ball.

4. Press dough into 9*9 baking dish.

5. Pour fresh raspberries and jam over the top of dough.

6. Take another bowl add flour, butter and sugar mix until it form crumbled mixture.

7. Spread crumbled mixture over the raspberries.

8.   Place baking tray in oven and bake for 35 minutes or until golden brown.

9.   Remove from oven cool for minute and cut into pieces and serve.

Nutritional Value (Amount per Serving):

- Calories 369
- Fat 5.0 g
- Saturated Fat 2.7 g
- Carbohydrates 79 g
- Sugar 42.1 g
- Protein 3.7 g
- Cholesterol 42 mg

Coconut Chickpea Soup

Serves: 6

Preparation Time: 45 minutes

Ingredients:

- 1 can coconut milk
- 4 cups vegetable stock
- 1/2 tablespoon coconut oil
- 1 zucchini, chopped
- 1 bunch of kale, chopped
- 2 carrots, peeled and chopped
- 1/3 cup red lentils, uncooked and rinsed
- 1/3 cup quinoa, uncooked and rinsed
- 1/4 teaspoon cumin
- 1/4 teaspoon turmeric powder
- 3 garlic cloves
- 1 can chickpeas
- 1/4 teaspoon coriander powder

Directions:

1. In sauce pan, heat oil over medium heat.

2. Add chickpeas, garlic, zucchini, carrots and kale in pan and cook until garlic becomes soften.

3. Now add turmeric, cumin and coriander powder stir and cook for 2 minutes.

4. Add red lentils, quinoa and vegetable stock and simmer for 15 minutes.

5.   After 15 minutes add coconut milk and simmer for 5 minutes.

6.   Serve hot and enjoy.

Nutritional Value (Amount per Serving):

- Calories 106
- Fat 1.9 g
- Saturated Fat 1.1 g
- Carbohydrates 16.2 g
- Sugar 1.8 g
- Protein 4.8 g
- Cholesterol 0 mg

Rosemary Lemon Chicken

Serves: 2

Preparation Time: 35 minutes

Ingredients:

- 2 chicken breast, boneless and skinless
- 1/2 tablespoon olive oil
- 1 lemon juice
- 1 teaspoon red chili flakes
- 1 garlic clove, minced
- 1 spring rosemary, chopped
- 1 tablespoon rosemary leaves
- 12 ounce small potatoes, halved
- Salt

Directions:

1. Preheat your oven at 450 F.

2. Cover the potatoes with cold water and salt in saucepan. Bring to boil potatoes over medium-high heat for 10 minutes. Drain and set aside.

3. In a bowl, place chicken and add spring rosemary, garlic, chili flakes, lemon juice, rosemary leaves and olive oil mix well.

4. In a pan, place chicken over medium-high heat for 5 minutes.

5. Transfer chicken in baking tray and add potatoes in tray.

6. Place tray in oven and roast chicken for 25 minutes.

7. Serve hot and enjoy.

Nutritional Value (Amount per Serving):

- Calories 438
- Fat 10.1 g
- Saturated Fat 0.7 g
- Carbohydrates 28.3 g
- Sugar 2.0 g
- Protein 54.3 g
- Cholesterol 142 mg

Roasted Potatoes with Garlic

Serves: 4

Preparation Time: 70 minutes

Ingredients:

- 1/4 cup Parmesan cheese, grated
- 4 garlic cloves, minced
- 24 ounce russet potatoes, peeled and halved
- 1 tablespoon butter
- 1 teaspoon red chili flakes
- 1 teaspoon Italian mix seasoning
- 1/4 cup olive oil
- 1/4 cup fresh parsley, chopped
- Pepper
- Salt

Directions:

1. Preheat your oven at 400 F. Grease baking dish with butter.

2. In bowl, add potatoes, olive oil, red chili flakes, Italian seasoning, garlic and cheese toss well until evenly coated.

3. Season potatoes with pepper and salt as per your taste.

4. Pour the potato mixture in baking dish and place in oven.

5. Roast potatoes in oven for 45 minutes.

6. Garnish potatoes with chopped parsley and serve.

Nutritional Value (Amount per Serving):

- Calories 257
- Fat 15.7 g Saturated Fat 3.7 g Carbohydrates 28 g
- Sugar 1.9 g Protein 3.2

Mix Berries Muffins

Serves: 8

Preparation Time: 45 minutes

Ingredients:

- 1 egg
- 1/2 cup low fat milk
- 2 cup whole wheat flour
- 1 1/2 mix berries, blueberry and raspberry
- 1/2 cup plain yogurt
- 1/2 cup maple syrup
- 1 tablespoon vanilla extract
- 1 tablespoon unsalted butter, melted
- 3/4 teaspoon baking soda
- 3/4 teaspoon baking powder
- 1/4 teaspoon salt

Directions:

1. Preheat oven at 350 F.

2. Spray muffin tray with non-stick cooking spray and set aside.

3. In a bowl, whisk together flour, baking soda, baking powder and salt.

4. In a large bowl, add egg, coconut oil, vanilla and butter whisk together until combined.

5. Add egg mixture, maple syrup and yogurt in dry ingredients and fold well until combined.

6. Now add mix berries in batter and fold gently.

7.   Pour the batter in muffin tray and place in oven bake muffins for 30 minutes.

8.   Cool muffin in the tray for 5 minutes before serving.

Nutritional Value (Amount per Serving):

- Calories 280
- Fat 3.6 g
- Saturated Fat 1.9 g
- Carbohydrates 52.1 g
- Sugar 18.6 g
- Protein 7.2 g
- Cholesterol 35 mg

Quick Peanut Butter Dip

Serves: 2

Preparation Time: 10 minutes

Ingredients:

- 3 tablespoon peanut butter, creamy
- 2 tablespoon honey
- 1 cup plain yogurt

Directions:

1. Stir peanut butter, honey and yogurt until well combined.

2. Serve with crackers and enjoy.

Nutritional Value (Amount per Serving):

- Calories 292
- Fat 13.6 g
- Saturated Fat 3.8 g
- Carbohydrates 30.6 g
- Sugar 28.1 g
- Protein 13 g
- Cholesterol 7 mg

Crust less Pumpkin Pie

Serves: 6

Preparation Time: 50 minutes

Ingredients:

- 3 eggs
- 2 cups can pumpkin
- 3 tablespoon all purpose flour
- 1 cup sugar
- 3/4 cup low fat milk
- 1/4 teaspoon ground cinnamon
- 1 teaspoon vanilla extract

Directions:

1. In a bowl, add flour, sugar and egg whisk together until well mix.

2. Stir in the vanilla, cinnamon, milk and pumpkin mix well until blended.

3. Pour batter in grease pie plate and place in oven.

4. Bake at 350 F for 45 minutes or until pie color becomes golden brown.

Nutritional Value (Amount per Serving):

- Calories 214
- Fat 2.8 g
- Saturated Fat 1.0 g
- Carbohydrates 44.6 g
- Sugar 37.8 g
- Protein 5.1 g

Healthy Banana Cookies

Serves: 6

Preparation Time: 25 minutes

Ingredients:

*   2 cups quick oats
*   1/4 cup low fat milk
*   4 ripe bananas
*   1/4 cup coconut shredded

Directions:

1. Preheat your oven at 350 F.

2. Spray baking tray with non-stick cooking spray and set aside.

3. In a bowl, mashed bananas. Then add oats, milk and coconut mix well until combined.

4. Spoon the cookie dough onto baking tray and bake cookies for 20 minutes or until it looks done.

Nutritional Value (Amount per Serving):

*   Calories 178
*   Fat 2.1 g
*   Saturated Fat 0 g
*   Carbohydrates 36.9 g
*   Sugar 10.4 g
*   Protein 4.8 g
*   Cholesterol 1 mg

Simple Baked Pears with Walnut

Serves: 4

Preparation Time: 35 minutes

Ingredients:

- 2 ripe pears
- 1/4 cup walnut, crushed
- 2 teaspoon honey
- 1/4 teaspoon ground cinnamon

Directions:

1. Preheat your oven at 350 F.

2. Cut pears in half and scoop out seeds and place pears on baking tray.

3. Sprinkle cinnamon over the top of pears.

4. Add walnuts on top of each pears and drizzle with honey over each pear.

5. Bake pears for 30 minutes.

6. Remove from oven let cool and serve.

Nutritional Value (Amount per Serving):

- Calories 120
- Fat 4.8 g
- Saturated Fat 0 g
- Carbohydrates 19.7 g
- Sugar 13.1 g
- Protein 2.3 g
- Cholesterol 0 mg

Egg less Mango Pudding

Serves: 8

Preparation Time: 45 minutes

Ingredients:

* 1/4 cup rice, rinsed
* 4 cups milk
* 1 teaspoon cardamom powder
* 2 tablespoon sugar
* 4 ripe mango puree
* 1 cup coconut milk

Directions:

1. In a saucepan, bring milk to boil over the medium-high heat.

2. Add rice in saucepan and cook for 30 minutes stir occasionally.

3. After 30 minutes add sugar and cardamom powder in pan and stir together until combined.

4. Turn off heat and let it cool. Layer rice in serving bowl.

5. Add mango puree and coconut milk in blender and blend until get smooth puree.

6. Layer this puree on top of rice.

7. Let the pudding chill in refrigerator for hours before serving.

Nutritional Value (Amount per Serving):

* Calories 162
* Fat 9.7 g Saturated Fat 7.8 g Carbohydrates 15.3 g
* Sugar 9.5 g Protein 5.1 g

Protein Chocolate Mousse

Serves: 4

Preparation Time: 15 minutes

Ingredients:

- 4 tablespoon coco powder
- 3 drop liquid stevia
- 16 ounce fat free cheese
- 1/4 teaspoon vanilla
- 2 tablespoon shredded chocolate

Directions:

1. In a bowl, add all ingredients except shredded chocolate and mix well until get creamy mixture.

2. Pour mixture in serving glasses and sprinkle shredded chocolate over the top of each glass.

3. Chilled mouse glasses in refrigerator before serving.

Nutritional Value (Amount per Serving):

- Calories 218
- Fat 3.2 g
- Saturated Fat 2.2 g
- Carbohydrates 19.4 g
- Sugar 13.5 g
- Protein 27.4 g
- Cholesterol 28 mg

Cucumber Salad

Serves: 6

Preparation Time: 10 minutes

Ingredients:

- 1/2 teaspoon olive oil
- 4 cups cucumber, sliced
- 1 teaspoon sesame seeds
- 1 teaspoon honey
- 1/4 cup vinegar
- 1/4 cup red pepper, diced
- 1/4 cup onion, sliced
- 1/4 teaspoon red chili flakes
- 1/2 teaspoon salt

Directions:

1. In a bowl, add sliced cucumber, pepper, sesame seeds and onion mix well until combined and set aside.

2. In small bowl, combine together vinegar, olive oil, honey, chili flakes and salt.

3. Pour vinegar mixture into the cucumber mixture and toss well.

4. Serve immediately and enjoy.

Nutritional Value (Amount per Serving):

- Calories 30
- Fat 0.8 g Saturated Fat 0 g Carbohydrates 4.4 g
- Sugar 2.5 g Protein 0.7

Avocado, Walnut and Kale Pasta

Serves: 4

Preparation Time: 20 minutes

Ingredients:

- 16 ounce packet pasta
- 1/2 cup olive oil
- 1 large avocado, mashed
- 1 cup walnuts
- 2 fresh lemon juice
- 4 garlic cloves
- 8 ounce bunch of kale, stemmed
- Salt

Directions:

1. Cook the pasta according to the directions of package. Drain well.

2. Add olive oil, avocado, walnut, lemon juice, garlic, kale and salt in blender and blend for minutes until get smooth.

3. Pour avocado and walnut mixture in pasta and toss well until evenly coated.

4. Serve warm and enjoy.

Nutritional Value (Amount per Serving):

- Calories 516
- Fat 52.1 g Saturated Fat 6.7 g
- Carbohydrates 8.4 g Sugar 0.6 g
- Protein 8.7 g

Roasted Veggies with Honey

Serves: 4

Preparation Time: 35 minutes

Ingredients:

- 2 shallots, quartered
- 8 ounce small potatoes
- 8 ounce carrots, cut into wedges
- 8 ounce Brussels sprouts, halved
- 1 tablespoon honey
- 2 tablespoon balsamic vinegar
- 3 tablespoon olive oil
- 1/2 teaspoon pepper
- 3/4 teaspoon salt

Directions:

1. Preheat your oven at 400 F.

2. Spray baking tray with non-stick cooking spray.

3. In a mixing bowl, add shallots, potatoes, carrots, Brussels sprouts, olive oil, honey, vinegar, pepper and salt. Toss well until evenly coated.

4. Transfer the vegetables onto baking tray and place the tray in oven.

5. Roast the vegetables for 30 minutes or until tender.

6. Serve immediately and enjoy.

Nutritional Value (Amount per Serving):

- Calories 195 Fat 10.8 g Saturated Fat 1.6 g Carbohydrates 24.2 g Sugar 9.0 g Protein 3.4 g

Baked Eggplant and Zucchini with Cheese

Serves: 6

Preparation Time: 50 minutes

Ingredients:

- 1 cup cherry tomatoes, halved
- 1 medium eggplant, sliced
- 1 tablespoon olive oil
- 4 garlic cloves, minced
- 3 medium zucchini, sliced
- 3 ounce Parmesan cheese, grated
- 1/4 cup parsley, chopped
- 1/4 cup basil, chopped
- 1/4 teaspoon pepper
- 1/4 teaspoon salt

Directions:

1. Preheat your oven at 350 F.
2. Spray baking dish with non-stick cooking spray.
3. In a mixing bowl, add chopped cherry tomatoes, eggplant, zucchini, olive oil, garlic, cheese, basil, pepper and salt toss well until combined.
4. Transfer the eggplant mixture onto the baking dish and place dish in oven.
5. Bake for 35 minutes or until vegetables are tender.
6. Garnish with chopped parsley and serve.

Nutritional Value (Amount per Serving):

- Calories 95
- Fat 3.5 g
- Saturated Fat 2.1 g
- Carbohydrates 10.4 g
- Sugar 4.8 g
- Protein 7.0 g
- Cholesterol 10 mg

Healthy Zucchini Hummus

Serves: 4

Preparation Time: 20 minutes

Ingredients:

- 4 zucchini, halved
- 1/4 cup cilantro, chopped
- 1 teaspoon cumin
- 3 tablespoon tahini
- 1 lemon juice
- 1 tablespoon olive oil
- 3 garlic cloves
- 1/4 teaspoon paprika
- Pepper
- Salt

Directions:

1. Place zucchini on grill and sprinkle with pepper and salt. Grilled zucchini for 10 minutes.

2. Add grilled zucchini, cilantro, cumin, tahini, lemon juice, olive oil, garlic, pepper and salt in blender and blend until smooth.

3. Pour the zucchini mixture in bowl and sprinkle paprika over the top of mixture.

Nutritional Value (Amount per Serving):

- Calories 134
- Fat 10.1 g
- Saturated Fat 1.4 g
- Carbohydrates 10.1 g
- Sugar 3.5 g
- Protein 4.5 g
- Cholesterol 0 mg

Mix Berry Quinoa Breakfast

Serves: 2

Preparation Time: 20 minutes

Ingredients:

- 1/2 cup quinoa
- 1/2 cup almond milk
- 1/2 cup water
- 1/4 teaspoon vanilla extract
- 1/2 teaspoon lemon juice
- 1 teaspoon cornstarch
- 2 tablespoon honey
- 1 cup frozen mix berries
- 2 tablespoon almonds flakes
- Pinch of salt

Directions:

1. In small pan, add mix berries, honey, cornstarch, lemon juice and vanilla extract bring to simmer for 5 minutes over the low heat.
2. In saucepan bring water, almond milk and salt to boil.
3. Add quinoa in saucepan and cover pan with lid and cook for 15 minutes over medium heat.
4. Divide cooked quinoa in two serving bowl.
5. Add mix berries mixture over the top of quinoa.
6. Sprinkle almonds flakes over the top of each bowl mixture.
7. Serve immediately and enjoy.

Nutritional Value (Amount per Serving):

- Calories 365
- Fat 16.9 g
- Saturated Fat 13 g
- Carbohydrates 49.1 g
- Sugar 19.4 g
- Protein 7.4 g
- Cholesterol 0 mg

Your Reviews are greatly appreciated, and your experiences help others cope with their own. Please do share your experiences, and help others.

More educational, & diet books on gout & inflammation that you may find helpful.

Search for them inside of Amazon.com

Join our Gout & Inflammation Relief newsletter.

Everything You Must Know About Gout

HR Research Alliance

Gout

The Ultimate Guide

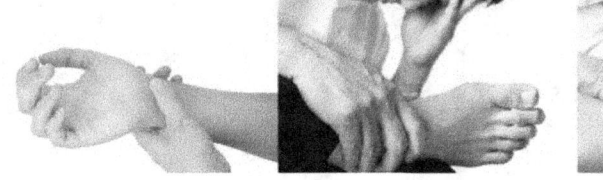
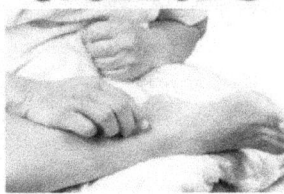

LIVE LIFE GOUT FREE!

GOUT REMEDIES ARE THROUGH DIET

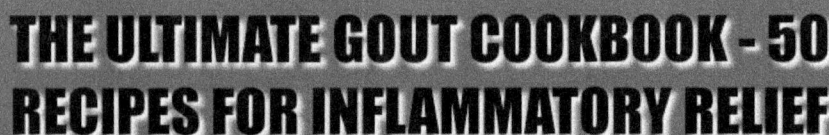

THE ULTIMATE GOUT COOKBOOK - 50 RECIPES FOR INFLAMMATORY RELIEF

GOUT BE GONE

HR RESEARCH ALLIANCE

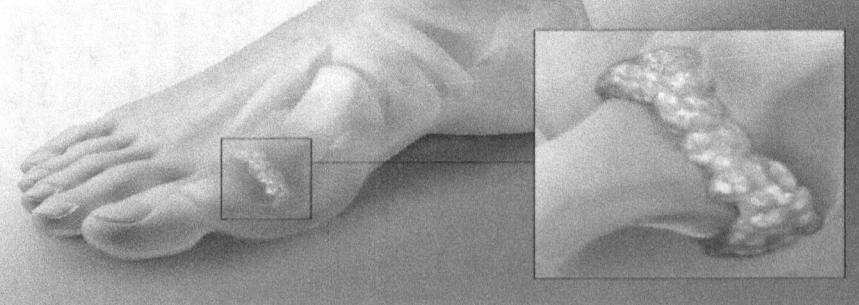

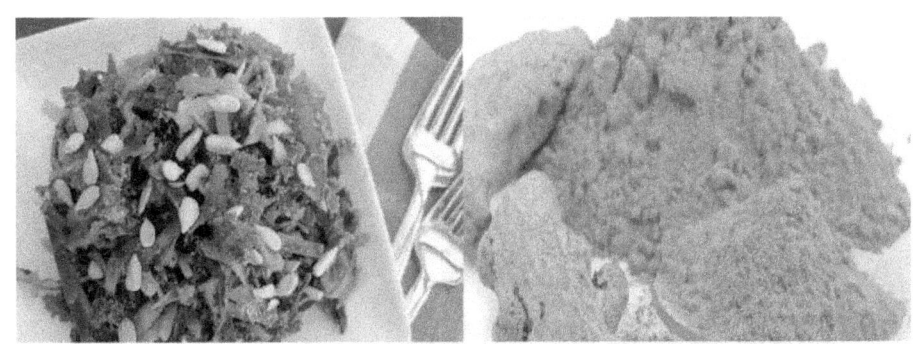

ANTI - INFLAMMATORY

COOKBOOK

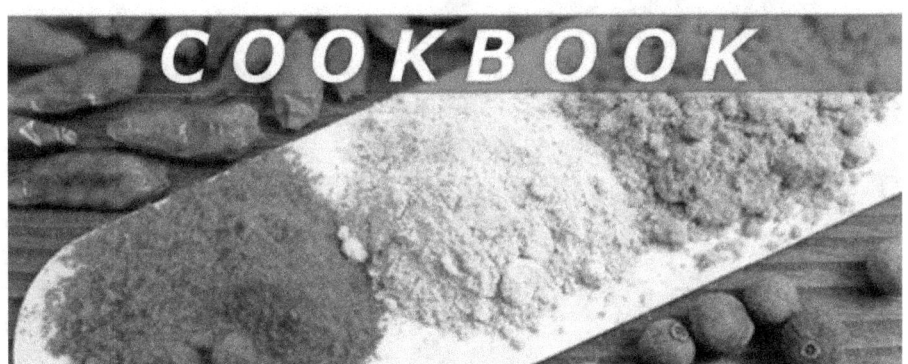

50 *Slow Cooker Recipes With Anti - Inflammatory Ingredients*

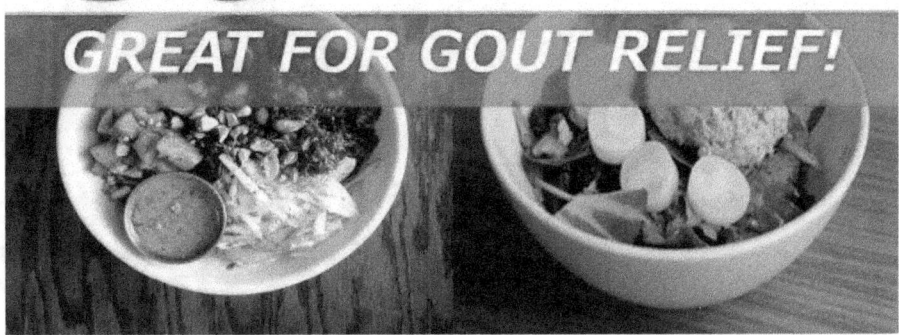

GREAT FOR GOUT RELIEF!

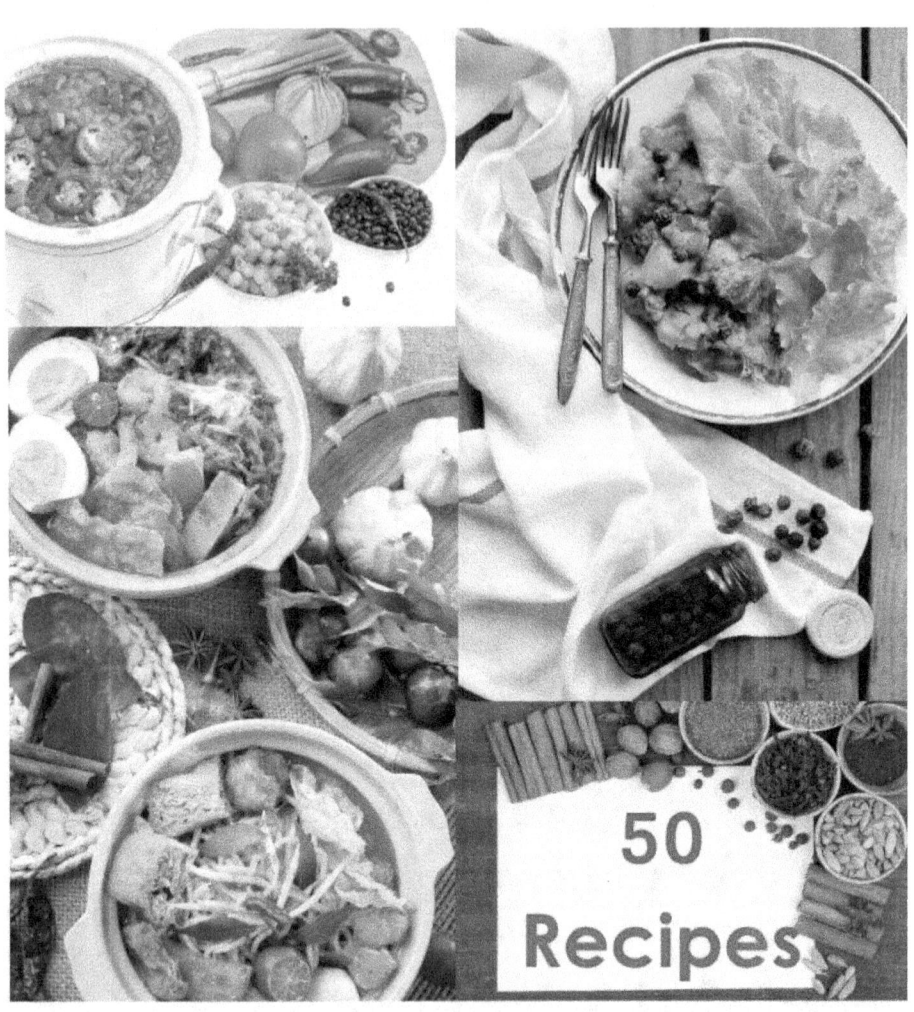

50
Recipes

GOUT RELIEF
RECIPES

Kelly Bird

Gout Treatment

Gout Diet

GOUT

Prevention

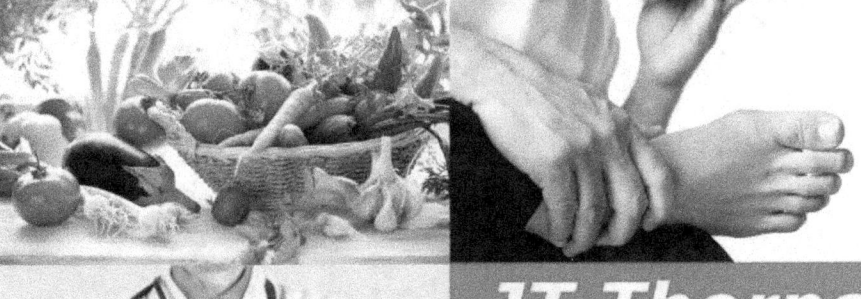

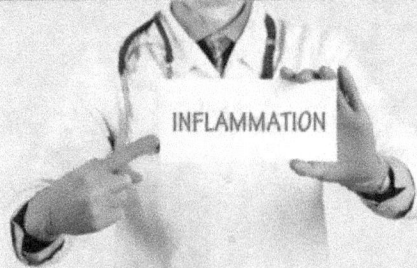

INFLAMMATION

Gout Relief

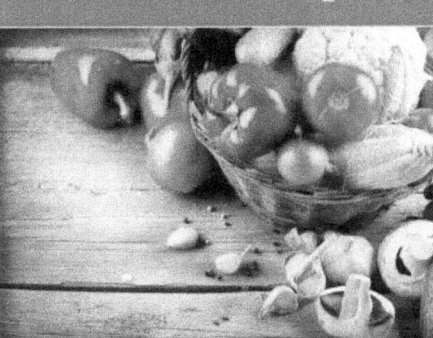

JT Thorpe

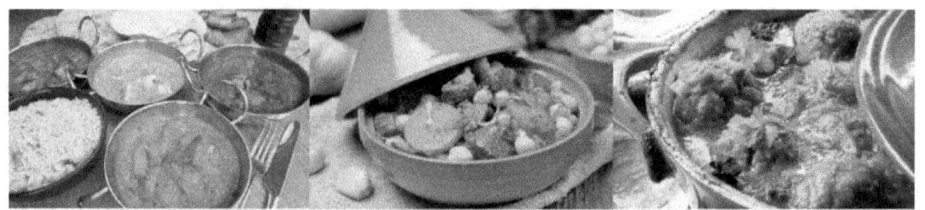

INFLAMMATION
Diet
Recipes

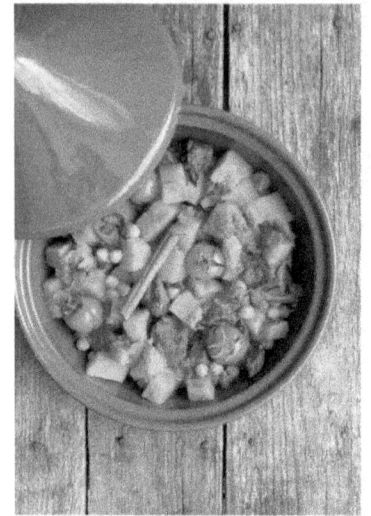

Great For Gout Relief!

70 Healthy Anti Inflammatory Crockpot & Slow Cooker Recipes

Cindy Myers

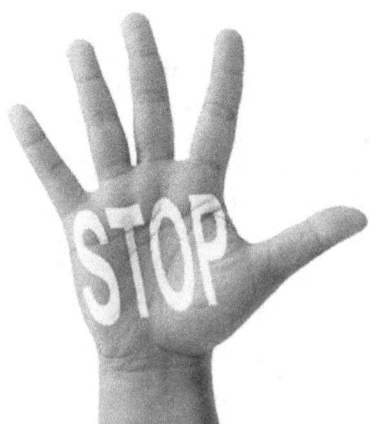

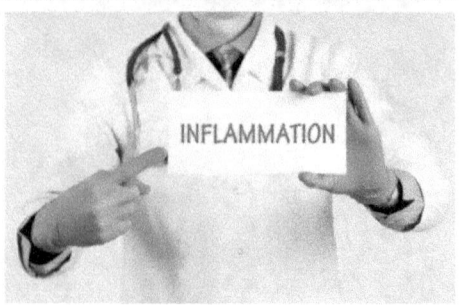

INFLAMMATION

www.ingramcontent.com/pod-product-compliance
Lightning Source LLC
Chambersburg PA
CBHW070152290526
45789CB00002B/735